NO MIND, NO PROBLEM

JACOB JI OGLETREE

Edited by
ALEX AURAND

To Ryokan,
for his one bowl and one robe

1

___

WHAT IS A PROBLEM?

___

problem

  ˈpräbləm/

  noun

    1. a matter or situation regarded as unwelcome or harmful and needing to be dealt with and overcome

___

___

"While meditating we are simply seeing what the mind has been doing all along."

— ALLAN LOKOS

___

One summer some years ago I attended a five day yoga and body tuning retreat with the humorous Glenn Black in upstate New York. One day in the middle of class, he said, "I can hear all your thoughts and they're disgusting. You all are offending me with your thinking.

Could you not think so much during class please? Thank you. Just imagine how much better off your life would be if you didn't think so much."

After class the idea of not thinking so much lingered with me. I knew he was making a joke yet at the same time, bestowing wisdom. I asked myself on the shaded path back to my dorm room what would happen to me in the absence of thinking. I stopped and took a deep breath, held it and slowly exhaled, looking around at the trees. My thinking mind had stopped and I realized that what really comes is the present moment, connection, contentment, fulfillment, and finally joy. I felt joy in the present moment, looking around in awe of the moment and being so intimately connected to it. I wasn't thinking of what had happened the other day or what I needed to think about to be prepared for the day ahead. It was a profound and simple moment for me, but eventually my present moment was broken with the sound of my stomach growling. I was hungry and then my mind went to what I wanted to eat for dinner.

To me, the idea of no mind seemed romantic, but not exactly practical for the everyday man. Still, I wanted to explore this "no mind" more. This pursuit ended up becoming a beautiful and transformative way to live my life, to experience more and more happiness, not only within myself, but to the outer world around me and everyone who crossed my path. I realized that my joy is the world's joy. Your peace is the world's peace. However, it still drew on a few counter intuitive notions of why we overthink and over-consume.

We *need* to think to some extent about things like planning out our day to day activities, making to-do lists, grocery lists, dreaming up the future, planning trips, logistical stuff, crunching numbers, weighing, measuring, etc. All of these types of thinking are useful and necessary. I found that in my case, however, I typically overthought most of the time. I believe the majority of readers will agree with me that they tend to overanalyze, overcomplicate and overthink things. We tend to project into the future or the past all the time. Luckily, there is a way out and you don't have to think to get there.

I wrote *No Mind, No Problem* to also address what the zen masters of the old days were always hinting at. *Zen*, or the state of Zen, is a state of being. Defining it, however, is a bit tricky. There are a lot of counter intuitive sayings about Zen. For instance, "if you are aiming for it, you are moving away from it; if you are not aiming for it, then you are moving toward it." It's all paradoxical and does funny things to your logical brain. It turns it off for a split second and sends the mind into a nondualistic state.

As nice as Zen is and as hypnotic an effect it can have when contemplating it, it is not very palatable to the average person who is balancing checkbooks and taking the kids to soccer practice. I wanted to make things a little less poetic and use keywords that wouldn't trigger one to say, "Oh, meditation. That's not for me."

I encountered this annoying wall of rejection with so many people early on and it frustrated me. I had family members who had never meditated in their lives. I almost gave up on the idea I could teach an old dog a new trick. When someone heard the words "meditation" or "zen" they were immediately turned off. Why? I don't know. I believe it could have to do with the association of the word to the audience. They probably visualize a Tibetan buddhist monk sitting like a statue and I can't blame them for thinking they were removed from it and that it looked too foreign to try.

I eventually learned to be more tactful and diplomatic

when teaching these things. I began replacing the trigger words with synonyms for meditation like, "breathing exercises" (because everyone can get behind the word exercise in the U.S.), "breathing consciously," "breathing mindfully," or simply "breathing." Even "consciously" and "mindful" were almost still too much of a stretch for some. I wanted the idea to be easily digestible and easily accessible to the point that I could teach meditation, zen, and mindfulness to any common man without him being immediately turned off.

You don't need to be a progressive liberal-minded Californian to be present. I became so much more fulfilled and happier by becoming more present. For years, I had the wrong approach to sharing the jewels of meditation. It left me puzzled, confused, frustrated, and even discouraged because a lot of people would just reject my attempts to introduce it to them. They rejected because of the stubbornness that often comes with not yet having experienced the joy and bliss of the present moment and also because I did not have the right approach to effectively show them that joy and bliss.

A painter of birds and a good friend of mine once handed me a book titled *One Bowl, One Robe: Poems by Ryokan*. I am not sure exactly why this book came into my hands, why she felt compelled to share the book with me. I think it left a more everlasting impression with me than it did her. The haikus and poems of Ryokan reached such depths in me and brought about moments of "no mind."

Ryokan was a hermit monk from Japan who lived in the 1700s-1800s. Of all the works of literature I've read of hermit monks, Ryokan probably speaks the clearest and touches my heart more than all the meditation masters. Ryokan lived a complete life dedicated to his monk-hood and the teachings and practices of the Buddha. He lived in an abandoned grass thatched hut on the side of a mountain, burned incense, wrote poetry, meditated, and begged for one bowl of rice most of his life. His poem "With No Mind" comes to mind as I write:

> *With no mind, flowers lure the butterfly;*
> *With no mind, the butterfly visits the blossoms.*
> *Yet when flowers bloom, the butterfly comes;*
> *When the butterfly comes, the flowers bloom.*

"So the Mind, So the Man" is another popular catch-phrase used in the law of attraction and manifestation circles that was originally a buddhist saying. I, too, actually used it in my previous book *Heavily Meditated: This is Your Brain on Meditation*. I talked a lot about the brain: about consciousness, the mind, matter, the evolution of the brain, what happens to the brain during meditation, neural oscillation, and how beneficial meditation is despite scientific scrutiny. It is fascinating, but also crucial in expanding one's horizon for a deeper appreciation and understanding not only of meditation, but of our own brain. The brain is something worth studying and trying to understand.

In this book, I want to address simply the essence of meditation, and not all the scientific data backing it. If I could boil it to a single sentence it would be this: we think too much and we spoil the present moment. That is the main message I want to share in this book. I have come to realize the truth: in spirituality you always add what you subtract. If you take more and more of the mind or thinking away, you will not only have fewer problems and worries, but more fulfillment and joy in this golden present.

When I set out to write *Heavily Meditated,* I spent six months locked away in a university's science library thumbing through neurological textbooks and looking up everything there was to know about the anatomy of the brain. I studied macro to micro, what science has to say about the study of meditation, the marriage of that science with what the traditional master meditators of the east had to say, and what their take on meditation was. That was all good and useful and I'm very proud of it, but I slowly realized that *Heavily Meditated* wasn't for everyone. It merely reached the halfway marker. I wanted to include everyone in this joy of the present moment, not just the fraction of the potential audience of serious meditators and Ted talkers. I wanted the most elegant and simplest of terms to use this time around in my writing to reach a wider audience and give them something useful, something very practical that everyone can enjoy and have access to.

2

WHY WE SUFFER

suffering

ˈsəf(ə)riNG/

noun

1. the state of undergoing pain, distress, or hardship

"If you want to conquer the anxiety of life, live in the moment, live in the breath."

— AMIT RAY

The untrained mind is like that of a child. It wants to grab shiny things, pick them up, hold them for one minute and then throw them away and start walking around looking for the next shiny thing to grab. It is constantly unsatisfied, grasping for this and that, seeking approval, acknowledgement, and attention, crying when something is taken away from it or when it doesn't get its way.

Do you know children like this? Do you perhaps know teenagers with the same capacity, the same self-centered mind? Do you also know some adults that act like this? We should not judge them or look down at them. To do so is to look down and judge ourselves, for they are a reflection of ourselves. The only judge is God.

People are usually not at fault for their untrained minds. When we understand why their mind is untrained, we can't help but have compassion in our hearts for them. The child often replicates and reenacts what it sees its mother and father do. Programming can come in numerous forms: culture, media, and society all play a role. Our fast-paced life takes a toll. Sometimes it's diet. A poor diet high in sugar can cause the mind to stay in a state of anxiousness. Sometimes it's a lack of mindfulness in the community.

If no one is there to teach how to water the seeds of the present moment and find fulfillment in the here and now, how can one be expected learn it? From a young age, we are pushed to act a certain way, think a certain way, and told we need to obtain certain things for happiness, security, and comfort. If no one is teaching us how to connect with our breath and body, then we go on living life in a state of ignorance and frustration. This in turn can breed mass disconnection to the present and mass ignorance. Only in the last 10 years or so have I seen more meditation classes being offered in schools to replace detention. It makes me very happy to see this taking place in the U.S.

The untrained mind leads to unnecessary suffering. If you look at Buddhism not as a religion, but as a methodology for the cessation of suffering, we can see that the root of suffering comes from within ourselves. We must train the mind with our breath to raise ourselves to use the higher faculties of our brain. When we can see clearly this image of our untrained mind, we can see how unnecessary suffering come from it. It comes in many shapes, sizes, and forms, from clinging onto things when it's nature is to ultimately change. The untrained mind is easily disturbed because its roots are shallow and can be pulled right out of the ground with two fingers.

When we cultivate our mind through breathing and mindfulness, we deepen our roots. Transformation is possible in the here and now. Nothing can uproot your peace, not even hell. When we first start to practice breathing in and out and become aware of this breathing, we will be pulled into the present moment. It feels so good to be in the present.

Much like anything else we attempt for the first time, it may seem difficult. So was walking, standing, riding a bike, speaking, reading. Mastery comes from repetition and consistency. It is natural to find something challenging or difficult the first time trying it. When you first sit, there will be a lot of commotion, clatter, and noise in your mind. You might be surprised to see how much there is when you finally sit still and breathe. Your brain will continue to be like that of a dog on a chain, barking and saying, "Let me off the chain!"

Your only duty is to just sit and monitor nothing else but your breath. All your thoughts will need time to settle. The mind eventually settles and becomes still and calm. You may be frustrated with getting quiet from your restless mind and constant thinking. This is natural. Your mind is like a circus. There are fierce lions, slithering snakes, cunning foxes, and wild monkeys. Keep the whip close and crack it loud. Until you gain self mastery over your mind, nothing else can be mastered or gained in this life, neither physical nor spiritual. With mastery of mind comes mastery of all things, even reality.

In life there will be pain. You may have heard the expression, "No pain, no gain," and it's true. To attempt to avoid pain or to anticipate pain is to suffer. Let it come and then let it go. There is a difference between pain and suffering. There is another saying, "Pain is inevitable but suffering is optional." You see, we do not have to suffer. It is our choice to suffer. We can choose to embrace our pain and transform it or to push it away and cause more suffering. Just walk with infinite optimism that every moment is new and that change can be made at will.

By training the mind through our breathing, all can be accomplished: peace, health, wealth. It just takes a little time. Lastly, the root of suffering comes not only from the untrained mind or lack of control over one's senses (what we taste, smell, hear, see, feel), but maybe most of all from selfishness. What it the best way to serve God while living in this world? By serving one and all. Don't ever lose a single opportunity to serve others. Serve, serve, serve and you will find that you are also served. Then there will be no more suffering, only joy.

Only in peace do we have joy. Not by acquiring things, not by doing things, not by earning or learning, but by dedication. Your entire life must be a sacrifice. Think for the sake of others. To such a person, peace is guaranteed.

You don't need to go to a monastery or sit in a cave somewhere for this — because it is not in renouncing actions that you will find peace, but in renouncing your attachment to the results of the actions. A truly dedicated person is the king of kings, the richest person in the world. Who is the richest person? The one who wants nothing.

There is only one cause for all worries and anxieties: selfishness. Restlessness of the mind is caused by disappointments. Only selfishness can cause unhappiness. To maintain your tranquility, you must keep your mind away from duality — pleasure, pain; profit, loss; praise, blame. If you can keep your mind away from duality, you can still have ideas and perform actions, but they won't affect you. When you renounce your attachment, there is nothing to shake you. It is the feeling of possession, of clinging, that disturbs the mind.

Test all your desires and actions. Ask yourself, "Is this going to cause restlessness to my mind?" Which should you choose: peace or that other thing? Peace is worth preserving more than anything else, even at the cost of your life. Peace is God.

Dedicate your life in the name of God, or humanity, and your mind will always be clean and calm. You will reflect your true nature always. That is the goal of all the different paths: to keep the mind clean and calm.

If you lose your peace, you won't be able to help anyone else, let alone yourself. Still, many people ask, "How can we do all these things for our own peace when the world is so full of suffering?" Normally, we think of the world first. But yoga teaches that the individual must be transformed before the world can be transformed. Whatever change we want to happen outside should happen within. If you walk in peace and express that peace in your very life, others will see you and learn something.

3

BIG MIND, BIG PROBLEM; LITTLE MIND, LITTLE PROBLEM; NO MIND, NO PROBLEM

ego

'ēgō/

noun

I. a person's sense of self-esteem or self-importance

"The word 'innocence' means a mind that is incapable of being hurt."

— JIDDU KRISHNAMURTI

If you have a big mind and a big ego, expect big problems. Everything will seem to be working against you or not in your favor. Your problems will be many and come frequently because of your big mind and big ego. I see people with simple minds having simple problems. I also see people with complex sophisticated minds having complex and sophisticated problems. Someone with a little mind will have little problems, a narrow mind, narrow problems, and the person with *no mind* has *no problems*. Do you see how your problems are going to fit the nature and state of your mind?

Even to the novice monk or beginner meditator, things will arise. That is because the mind is still there. An artist once said to me, "First I had to learn it all, then I had to unlearn it all, then mastery of my craft came."

It's funny how the mind works, isn't it? If, for instance, you are in a house of mirrors and you see your reflection in one of the distorted mirrors that makes you look very fat or pencil thin, wavy or in multiple places at once, do you become concerned and frightened? No. That is because you know that the *mirror* is distorted and not *you*. On the other hand, when we identify who we think we are with our minds, we take the state and condition of our mind or body to literally be us. If the mind is polished and shiny, we think *we* are polished and shiny. If the mind is dirty, we think *we* are dirty. Only when the mind is calm and serene can we see our true reflection in the calm lake of our mind's eye. Once we are calm and still, our true reflection will appear and we will see peace and serenity. Every desire and want is like throwing a stone in the still water and causing a disturbance in your peace. As long as you are consciously aware of these stones and enjoy the splashing then I say, "OK, enjoy it." If it is not serving you, stop throwing stones in the calm water and disturbing your peace.

Someone might come along and say, "You are so pretty." It can flatter you in an instant, especially if you are seeking the approval and attention or validation from an external source. The same statement can upset you if you think people only see you for your physical beauty and not for your intellectual beauty or spiritual beauty. It is all a matter of how your mind sees things, otherwise known as perception. Einstein discovered a great truth when he said, the universe is relative. Have heaven in your mind and you will see heaven everywhere. Then you are unbound and free no matter where you are. It's that simple.

If you live for today, in this very moment, and are content, all your daily needs will be met and you will be joyful, easeful, and peaceful. You will never get anxious over outcomes because you will be living a selfless life for others with the wisdom of having experienced your truth and your faith in a higher energy. Then we see that we are all just playing our part in the cosmic play, happily playing, unaffected by the outcome. This is what I have come to understand as truth.

The minute you put the mind, or ego, back into the equation, you run into lots of problems that your mind has created almost out of habit that prevent you from enjoying your life. It's really just you preventing yourself from your ease and peace. No one else. Your mind can say, "I don't have enough money" or "I don't live where I want to live" or "Once I get that thing, then I'll be happy," or "Look at that person, look how much health and wealth they have versus me." We create an ocean of division from experiencing unity, oneness, wholeness, completeness. In that state there is no longing, separation, or lack, but rather never-ending unity, happiness, and love. Abundance springs forth from our feelings. We can create either never-ending peace and happiness or a never-ending list of troubles, and conditions we think we need in order to be happy. The truth is that most of my problems and unnecessary suffering came from my attachment to people, places, and things. Even the things I always thought I wanted brought me suffering because once I had them, I realized they weren't what I wanted after all. My untrained mind made me believe I needed them more than I really needed them. Maybe you've felt similarly before. The times in my life when I was able to follow my heart and think less and just be are when I had the most fun, joy, peace, and bliss, and the least struggling, attachments, cares, worries, and problems. May you train your mind and reach heights of perfection within your own heart.

4

CULTIVATING FAITH

---

faith

faTH/

noun

1. complete trust or confidence in someone or something

"Trust in dreams, for in them is hidden the gate to eternity."

— Khalil Gibran

A mustard seed of faith can move mountains. Do you know how tiny a mustard seed is? It is so small. So why did they use the mustard seed as the analogy in the holy scripture? Because the smallest amount of faith can move mountains. Your faith is what makes you a believer. A true believer is someone who has blind faith.

The mind has a tendency to forget, that is why we call it the "mind." We have to "remind" it. The mind is fluid. It is not steady, but faith is permanent. Faith is a part of the true self. I used the analogy of a cloud to represent the mind. It moves in front of the sun and blocks the light. When it becomes concentrated, it is sometimes dark. Other times, it's white or thin. It is a continuously changing phenomenon. Don't get caught in the mind and its pranks. You rise above that. Just tell your mind, "I know what you are, I know you are mischievous sometimes, you are not going to pull me into this mud." Get outside of your mind and ride over the waves of your mind like a surfer. A good surfer doesn't get tossed by the waves, but rides them. The mind is nothing to be feared. It goes up and down and is just a part of nature, which is never permanent or steady. Even the atom doesn't stay still, but fluctuates. Just stand above the mind, watch it, and ride over it.

When you are learning to surf the small waves, they will frighten you. When you get good, however, you will start to look for big waves. A good surfer will not be happy with a small wave. He will say, "Look at that big calamity of a wave I faced today!" The mind can work wonders. Have faith and hope. Just think, "Healthy, healthy. Happy happy. Peaceful, peaceful. I will be all right. I will be all right. I will be all right." Then your mind will heal itself because all of our minds have that capacity.

How many of you have faith? How many don't? Everyone has faith, but faith in what? In something or in somebody? It doesn't matter who or what it is, as long as you have faith. Faith is important. Even God cannot help you, if you don't have faith, because your faith is God. Your faith is what you believe in. If you believe you are living, you are living. If you believe that you will die in five minutes, and you accept it, you will die. The doctors have even proved it.

Once, doctors made a patient believe that he would die by losing his blood, drop by drop. They had him sit blindfolded and made a small prick in his arm. He was told that his blood was dripping from his body into a bucket. He could hear the drops falling. When the drops stopped, the patient thought he lost all his blood, and he died; but, in fact, not even a single drop of blood had left his body.

We all live in faith. You have faith. You don't need to belong to any religion or "ism" or believe in any particular God. If you have faith, that becomes everything for you.

In South India, for example, the old women go to the backyard every morning and collect some cow dung. They take it to the front yard, stick a flower in it, and worship it as God. It becomes God to them. So, are they worshipping the cow dung or God? Because they believe that the cow dung is God, their faith makes the cow dung God.

We all have faith. Even if you don't believe in anything, you believe in not believing in anything. There's still a belief. Even a non-believer has a belief. You may not believe in what others do or say or believe in. You have your own belief, but know that you have faith and keep it up.

Now, you have faith in my answering the questions, right? Suppose I say, "no." Will you lose your faith? Accept it. Because there is an ultimate, higher will. God's will. Acceptance of God's will. That's the highest faith. Your faith in little things should help you raise up to the Supreme Faith.

5

TO LIVE WITHOUT PROBLEMS IS TO LIVE IN THE PRESENT

presence

'prezəns/

noun

1. the state or fact of existing, occurring, or being present in a place or thing

"Do not let the behavior of others destroy your inner peace."

— DALAI LAMA

King Solomon once said, "There is nothing new under the sun," and he was was right. There isn't anything that hasn't already been figured out by the yogis, mystics, saints, and sages. If we can realize this then we can start to relax more and rest easier knowing this simple fact.

All one needs to do is explore the holy texts of the illuminated beings and read what they say is necessary to experience the illumination of the holy word. It is not something that can easily be explained because it is to be experienced. I can explain what a blueberry is and what is tastes like, but you won't truly understand until you taste a blueberry for yourself. It is the same reading these texts.

I once heard that God is like the ocean. Man takes his boat out to sea, takes his bucket and scoops up the water and proclaims that his bucket is his understanding of God. Based on the size of the bucket, you will get a different concept and definition of God. Each person's bucket will be a different size based on the degree of their soul's evolution. (I think my bucket had a hole in it.) You can't capture God and bottle the infinite up.

I got very tired of church early on, not having experienced anything remotely similar to a spiritual experience. It's difficult to talk about God. You can only indirectly point at an aspect of His being. Someone can get behind a podium and preach about the Lord for five hours straight and have nothing substantial to say about God, because God is to be felt and not explained. You cannot put God into a bucket. You can only experience God as the ocean. It is better to jump into the ocean within your heart.

The truth is that you are the mirror image of God. You are already God. You are nothing less than God Himself. You are perfect in reflection. You are as pure and as loving as your creator. You are enough as you are, just as you are, whole and complete. You cannot be improved.

A lot of us in the west are busy sculpting and molding out our lives to look a certain way, so much so that we think we could actually make an improvement on ourselves. There is , however, an even greater sculptor at work who is going to mold us into something beyond comprehension. Why not give it a rest already, let go, and let God.

Your fears and worries do you no good. They are worthless, yet you continue to rent space in your mind to non-paying tenants. Why? There is only one reason: you are not present. Spend a little time with your life and your breathing. Connect your body and mind in the here and now. In this moment, do you feel that there is any lack or limitation? No. Here in the golden present, do you feel that you are in need of anything? No. You just smile because you are finally happy, and for no reason. Your happiness just IS. There need not be any reason. You have realized maybe for the first time or the millionth time that you *are* the personification of happiness. You accept life as divine perfection just by breathing in and out through the nose, feeling fulfilled and content.

Coming home to the breath and to the present moment is a lifelong practice. Will you become enlightened and remain ever in the present? I don't know, but that shouldn't stop us from coming home to our body and breath. You will continue to overthink and have unnecessary problems if you do not utilize the breath and pull yourself out of your mind and back into the present moment. Your master tool has always been with you and will always be the breath.

I could write a whole book on *prana*, which is your breath and life force energy. The breath is your master key to bringing you home to the present moment and connecting the body and the mind in the here and the now. Only then will you experience what it means to have no mind and no problems. You will unite the body and the mind and touch the miracle of life. Problems only come because of us. They are our own creations. It is in our lack of presence that problems arise.

Next time you catch yourself overthinking and feeling anxious, just take a step back, focus on the inhalation through the nostrils as you slowly inhale all the way to the top of your lungs. Hold the breath for a few seconds and then slowly let the air back out of your lungs through your nose or mouth incrementally. If you repeat this and focus your attention on the inhalations and exhalations, your mind will become very sublime and tranquil in about ten breaths.

There is such a thing as a presence "meter" or "road marker" that you can use to determine on average how present you are based on how much ease and bliss you are experiencing. If I've repeated myself in this book, it is because the message is simple, but crucial. Breath in, breath out, and smile. Breathe in and breathe out, focusing on the air coming out of the nostrils slowly. Be here right now! It's in the law of repetition; it needs to be repeated a thousand times until you start breathing mindfully more than once a day. Anyone can read a book on presence, happiness, and meditation. Anyone can do the breathing exercises in a book, but when the book is put down, how well have you learned? Did you take the book to heart? As one of my favorite living practitioners of mindfulness Thich Nhat Hanh says, "Breathing in, I am aware of this moment. Breathing out, precious moment. I pray that not only in my own life can I maintain my peace and happiness through mindful breathing and being present with what is." Om shanti shanti shanti.

6

———

PROBLEM FREE LIFE

---

freedom

ˈfrēdəm/

noun

1. the power or right to act, speak, or think as one wants without hindrance or restraint

---

"There are two mistakes one can make along the road to truth: not going all the way, and not starting."

— BUDDHA

I read a beautiful piece of wisdom recently: "When God wants to punish you, He will give you everything that you ask for." He gives you what you want, even though it may not be good for you. Unfortunately, we don't always know what we should want. We want many things, and a lot of those things bring us problems. So, in a way, we are the cause of our problems.

When someone has a problem, you might say, "Ahh, he asked for it." We don't necessarily ask for problems, but we don't really know what to ask for because we don't always know what's best for us. The best prayer would be: "God, I don't know what to ask for. I may even ask for the wrong thing because I'm still a child. As a good father, good mother, You know what is beneficial for me. You give me what I need. Please don't give me what I want. I will accept whatever You give me and I will accept what You take away from me. You are the giver, You are the taker." If you allow God to take things from you whenever He wants, you will never make a mistake in your life.

Our lives will be problem-free once we not only train the mind, but *master* the mind. You master the mind through the breath. I can say that sentence a million times and still will would not be able to stress this one point enough. By finding ourselves more present and connecting with our breath more, it can be the most fulfilling thing in this life and one of the most important things we can do as humans. It makes each of us a more finely tuned instrument in the hands of the Beloved.

There is a practical application to being present. We will act at optimal levels using the entire brain and our actions will be perfect reflections of our perfect presence. The ultimate goal of the entire world should be peace, despite our circumstances.

There are many people among us who still have untrained minds. It is an epidemic no one is talking about in this world and, as a result, the most scarce commodity is peace. You can't find it anywhere but right here and right now. Most people continue to run around seeking happiness outside of themselves and come up empty-handed. Love them and pray for them. In the end, you can only change yourself, but your peace is the whole world's peace. When you find the kingdom of heaven within and get a glimpse of His glory and joy, all other worldly desires will melt away and seem like a small flickering candle in the presence of the sun. Your whole life can be like this.

Everything is like a passing cloud. It comes, then it is here for a minute, then it is gone. Everything is always changing, always passing. If you can remember this, you can keep the ego small and just enjoy it all, the coming and the going. Once we achieve this level of acceptance and experience it through our breathing, we can no longer see anything but divine unity.

By continually focusing your attention on the breath, there can be no failure or disappointment or sorrow in your life. Hard to imagine, huh? Well, it's the truth. Don't be fooled into thinking you won't have to be attentive to your garden, constantly watering your present moment through breathing. Your practice is just like watering.

If a man should say that I am delusional or too lofty or not grounded, then let it be so, for if angels have wings, they reside in the clouds. My peace cannot be stolen, but man's gold and silver can. By focusing your attention on your inhales and exhales, you are constantly aware of the golden present; you are touching the miracle of life. Life is meant to be enjoyed. That is my prayer for you. May you breathe deeply and live fully in the here and now.

Your first and foremost duty is to find the kingdom of heaven within you. All the saints tell you to get back to the babyhood, the state of non-attachment. That is where you will find the kingdom. That is where all peace and joy come from. When you experience this, all the things you have been running after come out almost immediately. Name will come, fame will come, positions will come, money will come. Everything will be after you. There is a true greatness to one who renounces one's selfishness. If you are truly renounced and not running after anything, then intelligence and money will be at your feet.

All the knowledge and wisdom comes to you and sits at your feet because your mind is completely tranquil and balanced. You become a receiver of cosmic wisdom and, because you are not attached to it, it will come to attach itself to you. It is then your job to keep them and use them for the benefit of others. You keep them, but don't possess them. You have everything and, at the same time, you have nothing. You appear to be bound, but you are entirely free.

Only by raising yourself to that level do we have communion. What is communion? How do we communicate with God and have all the good qualities of God? How do you express God's love? You have to love unconditionally, never limiting your love. We have been given the freedom to choose right or wrong. If we want to communicate with God, we must develop this in our hearts.

God is one big transmitter, sending wavelengths equally to all. It doesn't discriminate between a rich man and a poor man. But who can receive these wavelengths? The ones who have receiving sets and who tune themselves to the station. You have to tune your meter to get the frequency and only then do you receive it.

God transmits His love in a cosmic way, on a cosmic frequency. If you want to receive it, you have to tune your heart to that frequency. You should become a cosmic person, an unlimited person. Don't limit yourself with your selfishness, but love all equally. When you remove all your limitations and become unlimited, then you receive God.

Every limitation is an impurity on life; every identity is an impurity. You rarely hear someone say, "I am all," but it would be a beneficial to think in this way. We should raise ourselves above all our limitations in order to become that unlimited and pure cohesiveness. When there is no impurity in your life, then people will call you a blessed person. In the Bible it says, "Blessed are the pure of heart." Why? Because only they can really see God. Why? Because God is pure and if you want to experience God, you have to be pure.

You should strive to be at the same level of purity as God. Unfortunately, we often try to bargain with God, "God I cannot come to your level of purity, can you come to my level of impurity?" God will come down and pick you up and walk with you. Everyone has their own name or idea of God, Allah, Krishna, Shiva, Jehovah, but despite the differences in name, we share the same higher power and should all strive to reach that level. We do, however, tend to try to bring that power down to our level because our limitations make it difficult to transcend. We even make God a human being, calling Him Father or Mother. You bring God to your level. That is why there are so many religions with a variety of names and forms of God, including different roles like master, server, child, father, friend, lover, beloved. Whatever relationship you want to have with God, just have a relationship with Him and aim to be as great as your idea of Him.

His willingness to have a relationship with you is an act of love. He is willing to lift you up as long as you are willing to change. We all have room to grow and improve. The only difference between effectively transcending and not transcending is your desire to change and your ability to make that change happen. God will welcome you with love.